Cure Painful Hip Flexors

Complete, Natural, Relief at Home

Your Free Gift

I wanted to show my appreciation that you support my work, so I've put together a free gift for you.

http://www.letoilepublishing.com/hips

Just visit the link above to download it now.

I know you will love this gift.

Thanks!

Introduction

If you are reading this book, then you are either currently living with hip pain or you know someone who is. Throughout the following chapters, I will attempt to educate you not only on how your hip works and reasons that it can begin to cause you pain but also on ways to alleviate that pain. It is my hope that by putting the techniques described in this book into practice, you (or your loved one) will not only be able to lead a more active, fulfilling, and pain free life but come to know that you don't need to live with hip pain!

Chapter 1: Living with Hip Pain

In this chapter, I will discuss what your hip is and how it works. I will also discuss exactly how hip pain can adversely affect your life and the lives of those around you.

Your hip has multiple parts that all work together to allow movement in your leg, which allows you to sit, walk, and run. Did you know that your hip consists of the hip bone, the acetabulum (socket), cartilage, and the largest bone in the body: your femur? In addition to the skeletal portion, you also have many tendons, ligaments, and muscles that come together at the hip, allowing you freedom (and control) of movement.

The most frequent cause of hip pain relates to the hip joint and not necessarily the hipbones. This ball-and-socket joint is one of the most used (and the largest) sockets in the body, and as such, is designed to withstand the stresses and pressure of long term repeated usage. Anytime you move your legs, you are using these sockets. Luckily, there is a cushion of cartilage, which keeps the friction to a minimum and allows for even, fluid joint movement.

However durable it may be, the hip joint is far from indestructible, and over the years the cartilage will eventually wear down or become damaged. The many muscles, as well as tendons, found in your upper leg can become overworked or strained. It is even possible for the hipbone itself to become cracked or broken. With all of the various moving parts in and around your hip, an occurrence causing your3 hip pain is not far beyond the realm of possibility. There are also non-injury related complications, which can be causing you pain. Ranging from a tipped pelvis to unequal leg length, the list of potential culprits is lengthy.

Living with constant pain of any kind, especially in high-use areas of your body, can completely change your life. It may limit your mobility or keep you from enjoying activities that you love. Pain can even affect the way your brain works! It can cause you to become irritable or easily agitated. If it is not managed appropriately, chronic pain may even result in the loss of a job, loss of friends, or in extreme cases, even divorce or loss of custody of your children!

It is evident that the pain you live with on a day-to-day basis can have many direct and indirect consequences, none of which are pleasant. Now that we know a little bit about how your hip is constructed and how it works, we can begin to discuss the various injuries and conditions that may be causing you pain and how to deal with them!

Chapter 2: Why Are my Hips Tight or why do They Hurt?

As mentioned in Chapter 1, there are many reasons why you may be living with hip pain. In this chapter, we will go over several of the various conditions and injuries that could be at the root of the problem. For ease of clarification, I will divide these causes into two groups: injury/disease related and non-injury/disease related. By doing so, we can narrow down the potential causes of your discomfort and better arm you with the tools needed to deal with your specific problem.

Injury/Disease Related Causes

Among the most common causes of hip pain is arthritis. Osteoarthritis, as well as rheumatoid arthritis, are found to be the most prevalent causes of hip pain (especially in the older population). By causing frequent inflammation in the joints, arthritis leads to cartilage break down. Cartilage's primary function is to cushion your joints. As cartilage wears down, or even disappears altogether, the pain associated with this disease continues to worsen. As the arthritis progresses, an individual may begin to notice a decrease in mobility due to reduced range of motion and may feel generalized stiffness in the affected areas. There will also be a degree of pain from the resultant inflammation.

Another major type of illness that causes chronic hip pain is cancer. There are several types of cancer that form tumors, which start in the bone or other that can spread to the bone. These can cause pain in your hips and may even lead to the necessity of hip replacement.

Avascular Necrosis is yet another medical condition, which is most often found in hip bones. Avascular Necrosis has many causes, ranging from injuries such as hip fractures or dislocations to long-term steroid use. This condition occurs when the blood supply to your hip bones is reduced, which causes necrosis (or death) of the bone tissue.

Conversely, bursitis, tendinitis, and muscular or tendon strains all originate from the same root cause: overuse. Both bursitis and tendinitis result from inflammation of the affected areas. Small sacks filled with fluid, known as bursae, protect our muscles and tendons. When we overwork our joints or are involved in repetitive actions that irritate the joints, these sacks often become inflamed and begin to cause the individual pain. It is much the same with tendinitis. Tendons are like thick rubber bands that attach your muscles to your bones. Overtime or with overuse, they they wear out and are prone to damage. Unfortunately, your tendons are not made of rubber. They are bands of thick tissue, which can become stretched or inflamed and begin to cause pain. Muscle and tendon strain occurs in a similar manner. If you overwork them by engaging in repetitive motions, this can potentially strain them, they may become torn, or may become stretched and inflamed, resulting in discomfort and potentially limiting your movement.

Non-injury/Disease Related Causes
In addition to various injury and disease related conditions causing hip pain, there are also several problems not caused

by injury or disease. I will not go into quite as much detail with these, as they are fairly commonly known.

One non-injury or disease related cause of hip pain is a tipped pelvis, which can lead to tightening of the hip muscles. Another cause is that your legs may be of unequal length, which causes both an uneven stance and an uneven gait. Both lead to overworking the muscles and causing muscle tightening or pain. Consequently, a common cause of hip pain is your stance (both standing or sitting). Leaning heavily to one side or the other may cause stress and pain on one or both sides. If your job requires that you sit for a majority of the day, after time, your hip flexors will begin to shorten. This muscle shortening causes hip, knee, and back pain while walking. You may sleep oddly or primarily on one side all night, which can, again, cause pain.

As you can see, there are many causes of hip pain. Take a look at your day-to-day activities and assess the way you sit and stand. Take a look at your shoes to see if there is uneven wear on the soles. This is a helpful way to see whether you lean too heavily to one side or walk unevenly.

Chapter 3: Let's Stretch!

As mentioned in the previous chapter, tightness in the hips is most often attributed to tightness in the hip flexors. Individuals with desk jobs are more likely to suffer from this as their hip flexors tend to shorten and tighten.

What exactly is a hip flexor and what is its function? The hip flexors are a group of muscles, which serve several purposes. Without them you would not be able to do such things as flexing the joints of your hip or raising up your knees. You would not be able to run, walk, or even crawl. Hip flexors are also responsible for the stabilization of your lower body.

Luckily, there is a simple way to remedy this problem. It is as simple as stretching to loosen the hip flexors and increase overall hip flexibility.

As a result, you have two choices: you can learn to live with the pain or you can choose to stretch. Luckily, stretching hip flexors has never killed anyone.

Of course, if you have worn cartilage or a cracked hip bone, the exercises contained in this chapter may increase your pain rather than decrease your pain, so, as always, consult your doctor before beginning any new exercise routine.

The Warm Up
Before you exercise, always warm-up to help prevent injury. The list of stretches includes, but is not limited too:

- **High knees**

Begin by standing with your feet hip-width apart. While walking or running in place, make exaggerated knee lifts, bringing your knee as high as you can toward your chest and alternating back and forth between legs. Start off slowly to reduce the likelihood of injury, and gradually increase the pace over the span of 1-2 minutes.

- **Leg swings**

There are two methods of leg swings to add to your warm-up routine: the forward leg swing and the side leg swing. For the forward leg swing, brace your body against a wall by holding out your arm to one side at approximately shoulder height. With both feet in line with your hips, slowly begin to swing one leg forward and then backward. Increase the height of the leg swing slowly until you have reached the maximum comfortable range. Do this for one minute and then turn, brace yourself, and repeat with the alternate leg. For the side swing variation, face the wall to brace yourself and slowly begin to sing your leg to the side and across your body. Then continue to build height until comfortable. Do this for one minute per leg.

- **Lunge with pulse**

To perform the lunge with pulse, start in an upright position. Step forward as if you were performing a standard lunge. The difference will become noticeable. Stop your lunge around one quarter to one half of the way down that you normally would. This is the starting point for the lunge with pulse. You will lunge up and down in short 3-4 inch increments each way, always staying in the lunge position and never returning to an upright position. Repeat as many times as you desire.

- **Walking Spiderman**

This next warm-up exercise is quite simple. Place yourself into a full plank position (body straight, arms extended) and begin to crawl in a forward direction by placing your right hand and left knee forward. Continue to move forward by alternating your arms and knees. Continue for one minute or your desired distance.

- **Lying Psoas March** (exercise band required)

This stretch achieves three purposes. Not only will it serve as an effective warm-up exercise, but it will help you put and keep your pelvis in a neutral posture, improving hip pain, as well as preventing back injury. The third purpose is that it will help you get rid of the "flat butt syndrome" typically caused by having a tilted pelvis.

To do the lying psoas march, you will need to lie flat on your back. Extend your right leg and lift your left leg up and bend

90 degrees. Take your exercise band and place it underneath your right foot, as well as over your left foot. Keeping your right leg in place, use your exercise band to pull your left leg forward bringing your left knee toward your chest while keeping your back flat against the floor. Hold this position for a moment, and then return your left leg back into the 90-degree position. Repeat this motion ten times, and then switch legs. Repeat the exercise ten times with each leg.

Now that you are warmed up and those hip flexors are ready to stretch, I will give you a few exercises to achieve the flexibility and pain relief. I also encourage you to look further for additional warm-up and stretches.

- **Butterfly stretch**

Sitting flat on the floor with legs outstretched, bring your right foot in towards your body; then do the same with your left foot. Your feet should be resting fully together. Bring your feet back as close to you as possible while remaining comfortable. Then lean forward as far as you can while remaining fully seated with feet together. Stop when you achieve a comfortable burn and feel your groin muscles stretching. Repeat this ten times.

- **The seated head to knee pose**

Sitting flat on the floor, place your right leg out in front of you. Put the bottom of your left foot flat against your thigh. Bend your right knee up so that you can wrap your hands around your right foot. Now place your forehead against your knees and slowly start to straighten your right leg while keeping your head as still as possible. Only use your arms to help keep your head's position. Keep your shoulders parallel to the floor while in the extended position. Hold this position for ten seconds and then release. Switch legs and repeat the exercise with the alternate leg.

- **Kneeling hip flexor stretch**

To perform this exercise, you will need to move onto the floor (or exercise mat) and rest your bottom on your heels with your toes planted on the mat. Now lean forward and place your palms on the mat, so you can support the weight of your body.

While lifting your left knee, rest your left foot on the floor and bend the knee to a 90-degree angle ensuring that the foot is directly underneath the knee. Ensure that your right foot and knee have not moved from their original position. Lift your hands off of the floor and move your torso into an upright position. Take your left hand and rest it on your left leg while placing your right hand upon your right hip. Doing this will give you stability while performing this exercise. You have now reached the starting position.

Now breath out and slowly move forward until you can feel the back of your thigh touching the back of your calf. Keep your abdominal muscles tight throughout these motions to keep your back straight and prevent possible injury. Hold this position, feeling the burn in your right upper thigh, for 30 seconds, remembering to breathe at a normal rate. Return to the starting position and switch legs. Repeat the exercise with the alternate leg.

Chapter 4: Self-Massage

Now that you have stretched and boosted your flexibility, you can transition into the exercise phase by practicing a little self-massage using a little spikey massage ball. This will make your hip flexors feel better by reducing muscle tension and regaining flexibility.

Lying stomach down on the floor, position the spikey ball underneath your hip flexors (between your pelvis and upper thigh). Resting on your elbows and forearms, use your arms and legs to move from one side to the other and from the front to the back, allowing the massage ball to effectively massage the hip flexors. Breathing normally, keep your legs and hips relaxed as you continue this movement for up to 90 seconds or as long as it remains comfortable to you.

Once completed, return to the starting position with the spikey ball on your hip flexor area and slowly bend your right knee and raise your leg off the floor. Straighten your leg and then lift it. Repeat this for up to 90 seconds, again making sure to cease if it begins to cause pain. Return the right leg to the floor and repeat the exercise with the left leg.

Once you have completed this short but simple step, you'll be ready to exercise those flexors! You will begin the process of making your muscles stronger to alleviate not only your current pain but also prevent future hip pain issues. Get ready to do work!

Chapter 5: Work It

So far we have learned how to warm-up the hip flexors. We have stretched them and massaged them to improve flexibility. We are now going to begin building up the strength of your flexors, strengthening them and increasing your mobility. Here are some exercises that work various areas of your hip muscles to achieve that goal:

- **Lateral squat**

While standing with your feet roughly twice your shoulder-width apart, lean to one side, shift your weight, and then bring your hips downward and to the back. Keep your knees and toes inline while holding your weight on the bent leg. Hold this position for 2-3 seconds and then ease back into the starting position. Shift your weight the other direction and repeat. Do this exercise in three sets of ten repetitions.

- **Four direction using a mini-band**

Put your mini-band at ankle height and place your feet approximately your shoulder-width apart. Keep your legs straight, and using your hips to create the motion, carefully walk backwards ten steps. Now walk forwards ten steps. After resting for a moment, take ten steps to the left, and finish by taking ten steps to the right.

You are now ready to raise the mini-band to thigh height and repeat this process. By altering the angle of resistance against your hip muscles, this allows you to exercise them differently and will enhance the overall workout.

- **Four way cable** (cable column and ankle cuff required)

For those with access to an exercise machine or cable column, this exercise will significantly help you build up your hip flexors. Be cautious. Start with a low weight and work your way up. If you find yourself leaning excessively to the side, you have gone too far. Reduce the weight. Attach your ankle cuff to the cable and attach the cuff to your leg. Being very careful to remain standing up straight, extend your leg slowly forward and hold for a three second count. Now return your leg to the neutral position. Extend your leg in the other three directions, holding each for three seconds before returning to neutral. Do this for ten repetitions and then remove the ankle cuff, turn, and attach the cuff to your other leg.

Now you've built a complete workout routine that will alleviate your hip pain (quite possibly lower back pain as well) and also prevent future hip and back injuries from occurring. Your posture will also be improved as a result of this routine, which is more important than you may realize.

Chapter 6: Stand up Straight

While walking down the street or into your friendly neighborhood mega-store, notice how people walk, stand, and even sit. You will likely notice that the overwhelming majority have horrible posture. They may have humped shoulders or hunched backs. They may have their head bent down looking at the ground. You might even find them sitting on a bench, sliding down in the seat, and bowing their lower back area. All of these postures can cause problems in overall condition, ranging from headaches to neck and shoulder or lower back pain to hip pain.

To alleviate all of those problems, we have established that overall good posture is important. What does that mean? What is good posture?

- **Good Posture**

All you have to do is stand up straight. That is it! Keep your back straight, your shoulders square, your head straight, your stomach tight, and your chest out. If you can accomplish this, then you are doing great. Picture a pencil drawing a line from your ear lobe, through your shoulder, down through your hip and knee, all the way through your ankle.

- **Standing posture**

Now that we have established overall proper posture, we need to equate that to good standing posture. Start off by standing with your feet approximately shoulder-width apart. Again, maintain good posture by keeping your head straight and your shoulders squared. Rest your weight on the balls of your feet instead of your heels. When you place your weight on your heels, you are more prone to slouching.

It may feel odd in the beginning, but your body adjusts from your old stance to the new one. To help with this adjustment, practice this posture while standing with your back to a wall. With your head, shoulders, and bottom touching the wall, maintain your stance. This will help, along with consistent posture habits, to train your body to fall into these postures normally.

- **Sitting posture**

Many of us sit at a machine or a desk for eight to twelve hours per day while we work. As previously mentioned, this of course wreaks havoc on your hip flexors and can also cause other complications if we do not make corrections.

If this pertains to you, when possible, have a comfortable, supportive, and ergonomic chair. If you are not in a position to make this dream a reality, bring a pillow or similar item specifically designed for lumbar support. Make sure you maintain good overall upper body posture, being careful not to slouch in your chair or lean over your desk excessively.

Keep your feet firmly on the ground and directly in front of you, and keep your chair adjusted so your elbows are at a 90-degree angle.

- **Walking posture**

Walking posture varies little from standing posture. The main difference is that you are in motion instead of remaining stationary. Keep your head straight. Most have a tendency to look at the ground while they walk. Whatever the reason, this pushes their head forward and bends the neck, affecting your entire posture.

- **Posture while lying down**

There are a few things you can do to help ensure good sleeping posture. Use a firm mattress, as soft ones do not generally provide ample back support. Try your best to sleep on your back. If you are a side sleeper, place a pillow between your knees and ankles. This pillow helps keep your body in proper alignment. Ensure that you use the right amount of pillows. Too many or too few can hurt your neck and cause you to not sleep well.

Chapter 7: The Daily Grind

Working to reduce or even eliminate your pain requires sacrifice. Is it worth it to you? Is it worth waking up an hour earlier to get rid of your pain? I suggest starting your day off right by maintaining all those postures we just discussed. Set your alarm clock earlier than normal, wake up, and give your hips some much-needed care.

Get ready by spending five minutes on your warm-ups. Spend the next five minutes building a repertoire with your spikey ball as you do your self-massage. The next 20 minutes belong to your exercises. Then you will have 30 minutes to enjoy a hot shower to prepare to face your day. Work for 30 minutes and then relax with a shower afterward, and you are on your way to a stronger, healthier, pain-free life.

If you have the desire and the willpower to repeat this routine daily for a month, it will become second nature to you and will no longer seem like a sacrifice of your time. It will simply be a part of your life. Over time, after the pain is gone, you may begin to evolve your routine into a more comprehensive workout, encompassing other areas of muscle groups. This will result in a better overall condition and improved health.

Chapter 8: That's all…Good Night!

We have walked you through a lifestyle change that will, hopefully, bring about a day when you no longer suffer from hip pain. We have discussed what your hip consists of and how it works, as well as how it deteriorates through age and excessive repetitive movements.

We have discussed the various diseases and injuries that may be responsible for your discomfort. You have discovered the importance of correct posture and how poor posture can lead to different complications, such as hip pain. We even discussed proper technique to stand, sit, and lie down. You were taught a series of warm-ups, stretches, and exercises, as well as reasoning behind each and doing them properly. These activities, when applied to your daily routine, can help to alleviate even the most stubborn hip flexor tightness.

We even discussed how to go about applying all of these techniques to your daily routine. The only thing left to do is do it.

Personally, as someone who lived with lower back and hip pain for over a decade, I can tell you firsthand how badly I wish someone had given me this information before it led to surgery. I wished for someone to tell me that once it gets to this point, I would never be completely pain free again. I cannot stress enough that if you are suffering from hip or lower back pain that is not due to injury or disease, follow the plan laid out in the chapters before you.

As previously mentioned, always check with your doctor before you start a new exercise routine. This is especially important if you suffer from a certain disease or injury that may be the root of the pain or are unsure what the problem is, avoid any possibility of incurring additional damage to the bone or musculature of your hip area. Watch your posture, wake up early, do your exercises, and take care of yourself. You will have a future free from hip pain.

Conclusion

If you or your beloved ones are suffering from hip pain, then the above chapters explain how to cope with it in your day-day life. The above e-book will help you understand how to react in certain situations and handle pain that can be unbearable. Daily exercising and maintaining correct posture, as mentioned in the chapters above, will make it easier to lead a more peaceful, fulfilling life.

Your Free Gift

I wanted to show my appreciation that you support my work, so I've put together a free gift for you.

http://www.letoilepublishing.com/hips

Just visit the link above to download it now.

I know you will love this gift.

Thanks!